# Building Great Strength

Easy exercises and routine to help build
inner strength and lively always

## Jeff Anderson

# TABLE OF CONTENT

# Chapter 1

**Understanding Inner Strength:**

**Foundations for Growth**

In the labyrinth of life, where challenges loom large and uncertainties abound, the beacon guiding us through the tumult is often the inner strength that resides within. This chapter serves as an illuminating journey into the very essence of that strength, unraveling its psychological and emotional intricacies to lay the groundwork for profound personal growth.

## Introduction: The Unseen Force Within

Inner strength, that intangible force residing deep within the core of our being, is the silent architect of resilience. Unlike physical strength, which is visibly manifested in muscles and might, inner strength operates in the realm of the unseen—the domain of our thoughts, emotions, and convictions. It is the steadfast companion that empowers us to confront adversity with unwavering courage.

## Exploring the Psychological Landscape

To comprehend the nature of inner strength, we embark on an exploration of the psychological terrain. Delve into the cognitive processes that underpin resilience, understanding how our thoughts shape our responses to challenges. Unpack the power of positive thinking, cognitive reframing, and the cultivation of a growth mindset as cornerstones of a robust psychological foundation.

## Emotions as Building Blocks

Emotions, the colorful palette of the human experience, play a pivotal role in constructing inner strength. Investigate the interplay between emotions and resilience, discovering how acknowledging and navigating feelings contributes to a more profound understanding of the self. From the depths of vulnerability springs the well of strength.

**The Tapestry of Well-being**

At the heart of this exploration lies the recognition that inner strength is not an isolated entity—it is interwoven with the fabric of our overall well-being. Discuss the symbiotic relationship between emotional resilience and physical health, emphasizing the holistic approach necessary for true, enduring strength.

## The Importance of Building Foundations

Why build inner strength? This section serves as a compass, pointing toward the significance of laying the foundations for growth. Inner strength is not merely a tool for crisis management but a guiding light that shapes our choices, enriches our relationships, and fortifies our journey towards a purposeful and fulfilled life.

## Navigating Life's Storms: The Role of Inner Strength

Life is a series of storms, and inner strength is the anchor that keeps us grounded when the winds howl and the waves threaten to overwhelm. Through anecdotes, case studies, and real-life examples, illustrate how individuals have harnessed their inner strength to navigate challenges, emerging not merely unscathed but transformed.

# Chapter 2

## Mind-Body Connection: The Key to Lasting Strength

In the intricate dance between mind and body lies the essence of enduring strength—a dynamic synergy that extends far beyond the confines of muscle and bone. This chapter is an exploration of the profound interconnection between mental and physical well-being, unveiling practical exercises and techniques that serve as a bridge, fostering a harmonious relationship between the mind and body.

## The Dance of Harmony: Unveiling the Mind-Body Connection

At the heart of lasting strength is the recognition that the mind and body are not isolated entities but intertwined components of a unified system. Dive into the scientific underpinnings of the mind-body connection, unraveling the profound impact each has on the other. From neurotransmitters to hormones, discover the biochemical symphony that orchestrates our overall well-being.

## Embracing Mindfulness: A Gateway to Self-Awareness

Central to understanding the mind-body connection is the practice of mindfulness—an ancient art reinvigorated in modern times. Examine the transformative power of being present in the moment, cultivating self-awareness, and attuning the mind to the subtle signals of the body. Through mindfulness, individuals learn to listen to their bodies, fostering a deeper understanding of their own physical and mental states.

## The Stress Response: Taming the Beast Within

In the cacophony of modern life, stress is a ubiquitous companion that threatens the delicate equilibrium of the mind-body connection. Explore the physiological and psychological implications of stress, delving into the body's response to pressure and tension. Equip readers with practical stress management techniques, ranging from deep-breathing exercises to meditation, empowering them to navigate life's challenges with grace.

## Embodied Strength: Physical Exercise for Mental Resilience

Physical exercise, often viewed through the lens of muscle development, takes on a new dimension when seen as a catalyst for mental resilience. Unveil a series of exercises that not only strengthen the body but also serve as vehicles for mental fortitude. From yoga poses that align the body and mind to aerobic exercises that elevate mood through endorphin release, readers will discover the transformative power of embodied strength.

## Holistic Nutrition: Fueling the Mind and Body Connection

The mind-body connection extends to the fuel we provide our bodies. Explore the role of nutrition in supporting both mental and physical health, emphasizing the importance of a balanced diet rich in essential nutrients. Delve into the impact of hydration, vitamins, and minerals on cognitive function, unveiling the potential for nutritional choices to enhance the mind-body connection.

## Sleep as Restoration: Nourishing the Mind-Body Nexus

In the realm of lasting strength, sleep emerges as a vital contributor to the mind-body connection. Investigate the restorative powers of sleep, examining its impact on cognitive function, emotional resilience, and physical recovery. Provide practical tips for improving sleep hygiene, ensuring that readers harness the rejuvenating potential of a good night's rest.

## Cultivating Mind-Body Rituals: A Blueprint for Balance

As the chapter unfolds, readers are guided in crafting personalized mind-body rituals—daily practices that synchronize mental and physical well-being. From morning mindfulness routines to evening relaxation exercises, these rituals become anchors in the ebb and flow of daily life, fostering a sustained, harmonious connection between mind and body.

# Chapter 3

## Building Habits for Resilience: A 30-Day Challenge

In the quest for enduring strength, the journey unfolds not in giant leaps but in intentional, consistent steps. This chapter introduces a transformative 30-day challenge, meticulously designed to guide readers through a series of easy-to-follow exercises and routines. Each day becomes a stepping stone, focusing on a specific facet of inner strength, ultimately laying the foundation for lasting positive habits that cultivate resilience.

**Day 1-5: Foundations of Mindfulness**

Embark on the challenge by immersing yourself in the practice of mindfulness. Each day, dedicate a few minutes to mindful breathing, observation, or meditation. Cultivate the art of being present in the moment, laying the groundwork for heightened self-awareness—a cornerstone of resilience.

**Day 6-10: Gratitude Journaling**

The power of gratitude transforms adversity into opportunity. For the next five days, establish a gratitude journal. Reflect on and document moments of appreciation each day, fostering a positive mindset. This simple practice becomes a powerful tool for reframing perspectives and building emotional resilience.

## Day 11-15: Affirmations for Empowerment

Words have the potential to shape our reality. Engage in the daily practice of positive affirmations. Craft statements that resonate with your inner strength and resilience. Repeat them daily to reinforce a positive self-narrative, fostering a mindset capable of overcoming challenges with unwavering confidence.

## Day 16-20: Physical Resilience through Exercise

Physical activity is a gateway to mental resilience. Incorporate a short workout routine into your daily schedule, focusing on exercises that engage both body and mind. From brisk walks to quick home workouts, these activities not only strengthen your physique but also fortify your mental endurance.

## Day 21-25: Mind-Body Connection Rituals

Deepen your understanding of the mind-body connection through daily rituals. Explore practices such as progressive muscle relaxation, stretching, or yoga. Each day, dedicate time to activities that foster harmony between your mental and physical well-being, nurturing a holistic approach to resilience.

**Day 26-30: Reflection and Integration**

As the 30-day challenge draws to a close, take time for reflection. Review your experiences, noting the changes in your mindset and overall well-being. Identify the exercises and routines that resonated most with you. Integrate these practices into your daily life, transforming them from a challenge into enduring habits that fortify your resilience.

# Chapter 4

**The Power of Positive Affirmations: Rewiring Your Mind for Strength**

In the intricate tapestry of the mind, the threads of our thoughts weave the narrative of our daily lives. This chapter delves into the transformative realm of positive affirmations—a potent tool for reshaping the narrative and cultivating mental strength. As we explore the impact of affirmations, we will present a collection of powerful statements and guide readers on the art of integrating them into their daily routines to foster a positive mindset capable of overcoming challenges with resilience and fortitude.

## Understanding Affirmations: Seeds of Empowerment

Affirmations are more than mere words; they are seeds planted in the fertile soil of the mind. Uncover the psychological mechanisms that underpin the effectiveness of affirmations, exploring how they influence thought patterns, beliefs, and ultimately, behavior. Learn how the mind's receptivity to positive statements can pave the way for a profound shift in mindset.

**Crafting Powerful Affirmations: Words That Resonate**

Present readers with a curated collection of powerful affirmations that resonate with the themes of resilience, inner strength, and empowerment. These statements serve as beacons of positivity, guiding individuals through moments of self-doubt and adversity. Encourage readers to select or adapt affirmations that align with their personal aspirations and challenges.

## Integrating Affirmations into Daily Life: A Ritual of Reinforcement

Guide readers in establishing a daily ritual for affirmations. Whether through morning reflections, midday resets, or evening affirmations, provide practical tips on when and how to incorporate these powerful statements into their routine. Emphasize the importance of consistency to harness the cumulative effect of positive reinforcement.

## Overcoming Negative Self-Talk: Affirmations as a Shield

Explore the insidious nature of negative self-talk and how affirmations serve as a shield against its corrosive influence. Equip readers with strategies to identify and counteract self-limiting beliefs, fostering a mindset that is resilient in the face of challenges. Affirmations become a tool for rewriting the narrative of self-doubt.

## The Neuroscience of Affirmations: Rewiring Neural Pathways

Delve into the neuroscience behind affirmations, unraveling how these positive statements have the power to rewire neural pathways. Explore the concept of neuroplasticity and how consistent affirmation practices can create lasting changes in the brain, reinforcing a positive and resilient mindset.

## Affirmations in Times of Challenge: A Guiding Light

Examine the role of affirmations during moments of adversity. Illustrate how affirmations can be a guiding light, providing solace, motivation, and clarity when faced with life's inevitable challenges. Share real-life examples of individuals who have navigated difficulties with the support of positive affirmations.

**Personalizing Affirmations: A Journey of Self-Discovery**

Encourage readers to personalize affirmations based on their unique strengths, values, and goals. Provide guidance on crafting affirmations that resonate authentically, reflecting the individual's journey toward greater resilience and inner strength. This personal touch enhances the efficacy of affirmations in fostering a positive mindset.

# Chapter 5

## Lively Always: Energizing Exercises for a Vibrant Life

In the rhythmic dance of life, vitality is the melody that propels us forward. This chapter is an invitation to embrace a lively and active lifestyle through a curated collection of energizing exercises. Designed to be simple yet effective, these activities incorporate elements of yoga, stretching, and quick workouts, offering a holistic approach to boosting energy levels and infusing life with vibrancy.

## The Importance of Daily Movement: Fueling the Energy Reservoir

Unlock the door to a vibrant life by exploring the fundamental role of daily movement in sustaining energy levels. Delve into the benefits of exercise on physical and mental well-being, laying the groundwork for a dynamic routine that energizes the body and invigorates the mind.

## Morning Wake-Up Routine: Energizing the Body and Mind

Introduce readers to a series of morning exercises designed to kickstart the day with vitality. From dynamic stretches to invigorating yoga poses, create a routine that energizes muscles, enhances flexibility, and sets a positive tone for the day ahead. These exercises become a cornerstone for a lively and productive morning routine.

## Desk Energizers: Revitalizing the Workday

Incorporate energizing exercises that can be seamlessly woven into a busy workday. Share quick desk stretches, breathing exercises, and seated yoga poses to combat the sedentary nature of office life. These exercises serve as a remedy for fatigue, promoting sustained focus and productivity.

## Afternoon Pick-Me-Ups: Recharge with Quick Workouts

Guide readers through a repertoire of quick, high-energy workouts suitable for the afternoon slump. These exercises, ranging from brisk walks to bodyweight workouts, provide a burst of energy, combatting fatigue and revitalizing the body and mind. Say goodbye to lethargy and embrace an active, lively lifestyle.

## Yoga for Energy: Flowing Movements and Deep Breaths

Explore the rejuvenating power of yoga as a means to enhance energy levels. Present a series of yoga sequences that focus on flowing movements, deep breathing, and mindful awareness. Yoga becomes not only a physical exercise but a holistic practice that nourishes the body, mind, and spirit.

## Evening Unwind: Relaxation Exercises for Renewed Energy

As the day winds down, transition into a set of relaxation exercises that prepare the body for restorative sleep. From gentle stretches to calming breathwork, these exercises help release tension, promoting relaxation and ensuring a rejuvenated start to the next day.

**Weekend Adventures: Outdoor Activities for Vitality**

Encourage readers to infuse their weekends with outdoor activities that elevate heart rates and stimulate energy levels. From hiking and cycling to outdoor yoga sessions, these adventures become opportunities to embrace nature, rejuvenate the senses, and foster a lively and adventurous spirit.

**Creating Lasting Habits: Integrating Energy-Boosting Exercises**

Conclude the chapter by guiding readers on how to integrate these exercises into their daily lives. Provide tips on building habits that promote a lively and active lifestyle, emphasizing the transformative impact of consistency on overall vitality.

# Chapter 6

## Nutrition for Inner Strength: Fueling Your Body and Mind

In the intricate tapestry of inner strength, the threads of nutrition weave a foundational role in crafting resilience and vitality. This chapter delves into the crucial role of nutrition, offering a panoramic view of how food choices influence both physical and mental well-being. Practical advice on adopting a balanced and nourishing diet becomes the cornerstone, enhancing the efficacy of strength-building exercises and fortifying the body and mind.

**Understanding the Nutritional Tapestry**

Embark on a journey into the nutritional landscape, unraveling the interplay between food and inner strength. Explore the macronutrients and micronutrients essential for sustaining physical and mental well-being. The chapter sets the stage for the recognition that food is not merely fuel but a powerful contributor to the holistic strength-building journey.

## Balanced Diets: The Cornerstone of Inner Strength

Highlight the significance of a balanced diet in fostering inner strength. Emphasize the importance of incorporating a variety of foods, including fruits, vegetables, whole grains, lean proteins, and healthy fats. This diverse approach ensures a comprehensive range of nutrients that support physical resilience and mental clarity.

## Hydration for Vigor: The Overlooked Elixir

Dive into the often underestimated role of hydration in building inner strength. Explore the impact of water on cognitive function, physical performance, and emotional well-being. Provide practical tips for ensuring adequate hydration, enhancing the body's ability to perform optimally in strength-building exercises.

## Mindful Eating: A Ritual for Nourishment

Introduce the concept of mindful eating as a practice that transcends the act of consuming food. Guide readers in cultivating awareness around their eating habits, savoring each bite, and recognizing the connection between food choices and emotional well-being. Mindful eating becomes a transformative ritual for nourishing both the body and the mind.

**Superfoods for Inner Strength: A Nutrient-Packed Arsenal**

Present a selection of nutrient-dense superfoods that serve as powerhouses for inner strength. From omega-3 fatty acids found in fatty fish to antioxidants in berries, these superfoods provide a concentrated source of nutrients that support cognitive function, boost energy levels, and enhance overall resilience.

**Fueling Workouts: Pre- and Post-Exercise Nutrition**

Explore the symbiotic relationship between nutrition and exercise, focusing on the importance of pre- and post-workout nutrition. Provide practical guidance on fueling the body before exercise to optimize performance and replenishing nutrients afterward to support recovery. This strategic approach maximizes the benefits of strength-building exercises.

**Nutrition for Mental Resilience: The Gut-Brain Connection**

Delve into the fascinating realm of the gut-brain connection, uncovering how the microbiome influences mental health and resilience. Discuss the impact of probiotics and prebiotics on mood regulation and stress response, emphasizing the role of nutrition in nurturing a healthy gut for a resilient mind.

**Creating Sustainable Habits: The Nutrition-Exercise Synergy**

Conclude the chapter by guiding readers on how to integrate nutritional principles into their daily lives, seamlessly aligning with strength-building exercises. Offer practical tips for meal planning, mindful grocery shopping, and maintaining a balanced diet that becomes a sustainable and enriching lifestyle.

# Chapter 7

## Overcoming Mental Barriers: Breaking Through Limiting Beliefs

In the pursuit of inner strength, the greatest obstacles often arise not from external challenges, but from within the recesses of our own minds. This chapter is an exploration of the mental barriers that impede the development of resilience and empowerment. By identifying these limiting beliefs and offering practical strategies and exercises, readers will be equipped to break through these barriers, fostering a transformative mindset of growth and empowerment.

**Unmasking Limiting Beliefs: The Chains Within**

Begin by unveiling the common mental barriers that shackle the spirit and hinder inner strength. Whether born from self-doubt, fear of failure, or societal expectations, these limiting beliefs manifest as internal roadblocks.

Acknowledge their existence as the first step toward dismantling their influence.

## The Power of Self-Reflection: Illuminating Shadows

Guide readers through self-reflection exercises to unearth their own limiting beliefs. Through journaling, mindfulness, and introspection, individuals can identify the deeply ingrained thoughts that may be holding them back. This process sets the stage for conscious awareness and targeted intervention.

## Cognitive Restructuring: Rewiring Thought Patterns

Introduce the concept of cognitive restructuring as a powerful tool for breaking through limiting beliefs. Provide exercises that guide readers in challenging negative thought patterns and replacing them with empowering, constructive thoughts. This reshaping of cognitive landscapes forms the foundation for a mindset conducive to inner strength.

## Affirmations as Catalysts: Reinforcing Positive Beliefs

Building upon the earlier exploration of positive affirmations, emphasize their role as catalysts for overcoming limiting beliefs. Offer specific affirmations tailored to address common mental barriers. Encourage readers to integrate these affirmations into their daily routines, reinforcing a positive narrative that counteracts self-imposed limitations.

**Fear as a Guide: Transforming Challenges into Growth Opportunities**

Examine the role of fear in perpetuating limiting beliefs and reframing it as a guide for growth. Illustrate how facing fears, rather than avoiding them, can be a transformative experience. Share stories of individuals who embraced discomfort, transcending their limiting beliefs to achieve newfound strength and resilience.

## Mindfulness Meditation: Breaking Free from Mental Chains

Explore mindfulness meditation as a practice for breaking free from the chains of limiting beliefs. Through guided meditation exercises, readers learn to observe their thoughts without judgment, creating space for awareness and intentional mindset shifts. Mindfulness becomes a powerful ally in the journey toward inner strength.

## Constructive Self-Talk: Shaping Empowering Narratives

Highlight the impact of self-talk on mindset and resilience. Provide strategies for cultivating constructive self-talk by reframing negative thoughts and emphasizing one's strengths and capabilities. Through consistent practice, readers learn to reshape the internal dialogue, fostering a mindset that thrives on challenges rather than succumbing to limitations.

**Building a Supportive Environment: Allies on the Journey**

Discuss the importance of surrounding oneself with a supportive environment. Whether through positive relationships, mentors, or communities that share similar goals, having allies on the journey can be instrumental in overcoming mental barriers. Connection becomes a source of strength and encouragement.

# Chapter 8

## Building Lasting Strength: Long-Term Strategies for a Resilient Life

As we embark on the culmination of our journey toward inner strength, this chapter serves as a compass, distilling the key principles and practices unveiled throughout the book. It is a blueprint for building lasting strength—a roadmap for integrating these strategies into a long-term lifestyle that cultivates sustained resilience. Emphasis is placed on the twin pillars of consistency and adaptation, acknowledging their role in navigating life's ever-evolving challenges.

## Foundations Revisited: A Recap of Inner Strength

Begin by revisiting the core principles of inner strength, emphasizing the interconnected nature of physical and mental well-being. Reflect on the importance of understanding, embracing mindfulness, and fostering a mindset of growth and empowerment as foundational elements.

## Habitual Harmony: The 30-Day Challenge as a Launchpad

Recall the transformative 30-day challenge introduced in Chapter 3, recognizing it not as a mere exercise but as a launchpad for lasting habits. Reiterate the significance of incorporating mindfulness, gratitude, positive affirmations, and physical activity into daily life, creating a harmonious routine that fortifies inner strength.

## Mind-Body Mastery: The Key to Lasting Strength

Revisit the exploration of the mind-body connection in Chapter 2, underscoring its importance in sustaining lasting strength. Encourage readers to continue the practices that harmonize mental and physical well-being, recognizing the ongoing interplay between thoughts and bodily vitality.

## Affirmations as Daily Allies: Rewiring the Mind Continuously

Echo the power of positive affirmations introduced in Chapter 4 as daily allies in the journey of building inner strength. Remind readers to weave these affirmations into their ongoing narrative, using them as a tool for consistently rewiring the mind for resilience, optimism, and empowerment.

## Energizing Rituals: A Vibrant Lifestyle Unveiled

Recapture the lively exercises introduced in Chapter 5, framing them not as occasional activities but as vibrant rituals woven into the fabric of daily life. Highlight the transformative impact of consistent physical activity on energy levels, vitality, and the overall quality of life.

## Nutritional Wisdom: Fueling the Fire Within

Reiterate the nutritional principles discussed in Chapter 6, emphasizing the role of balanced and mindful eating as a sustained practice. Guide readers in making informed choices that nourish both body and mind, recognizing nutrition as an enduring foundation for inner strength.

## Mental Freedom: Breaking Through Limitations

Review the strategies for overcoming mental barriers explored in Chapter 7. Reemphasize the importance of self-reflection, cognitive restructuring, and cultivating a growth mindset. Encourage readers to continuously confront and break through their limiting beliefs, fostering mental freedom as an ongoing practice.

## Adaptability as a Superpower: Navigating Life's Changes

Highlight the inherent adaptability introduced throughout the book as a superpower in the journey toward lasting strength. Acknowledge that life is dynamic, and resilience lies in the ability to adapt to changing circumstances. Provide guidance on cultivating adaptability as a cornerstone for sustained inner strength.

**Consistency and Evolution: The Twin Pillars of Resilience**

Conclude by emphasizing the twin pillars of consistency and adaptation. Stress the importance of maintaining consistent practices while also being open to evolution and refinement. In this delicate balance, resilience flourishes, and inner strength becomes an enduring force capable of weathering life's storms.

## Conclusion: A Life of Resilient Flourishing

As you conclude this chapter and, by extension, the book, you are invited to envision a life of resilient flourishing—a life where inner strength is not a fleeting achievement but an ever-evolving journey. The strategies, principles, and practices discussed serve as lifelong companions, guiding individuals toward a future characterized by sustained resilience, enduring strength, and an unwavering capacity to thrive in the face of life's complexities. The journey toward lasting strength is not finite; it is a perpetual quest, an odyssey of self-discovery, growth, and the continual cultivation of an empowered and resilient existence.